PCP:

HIGH RISK ON THE STREETS

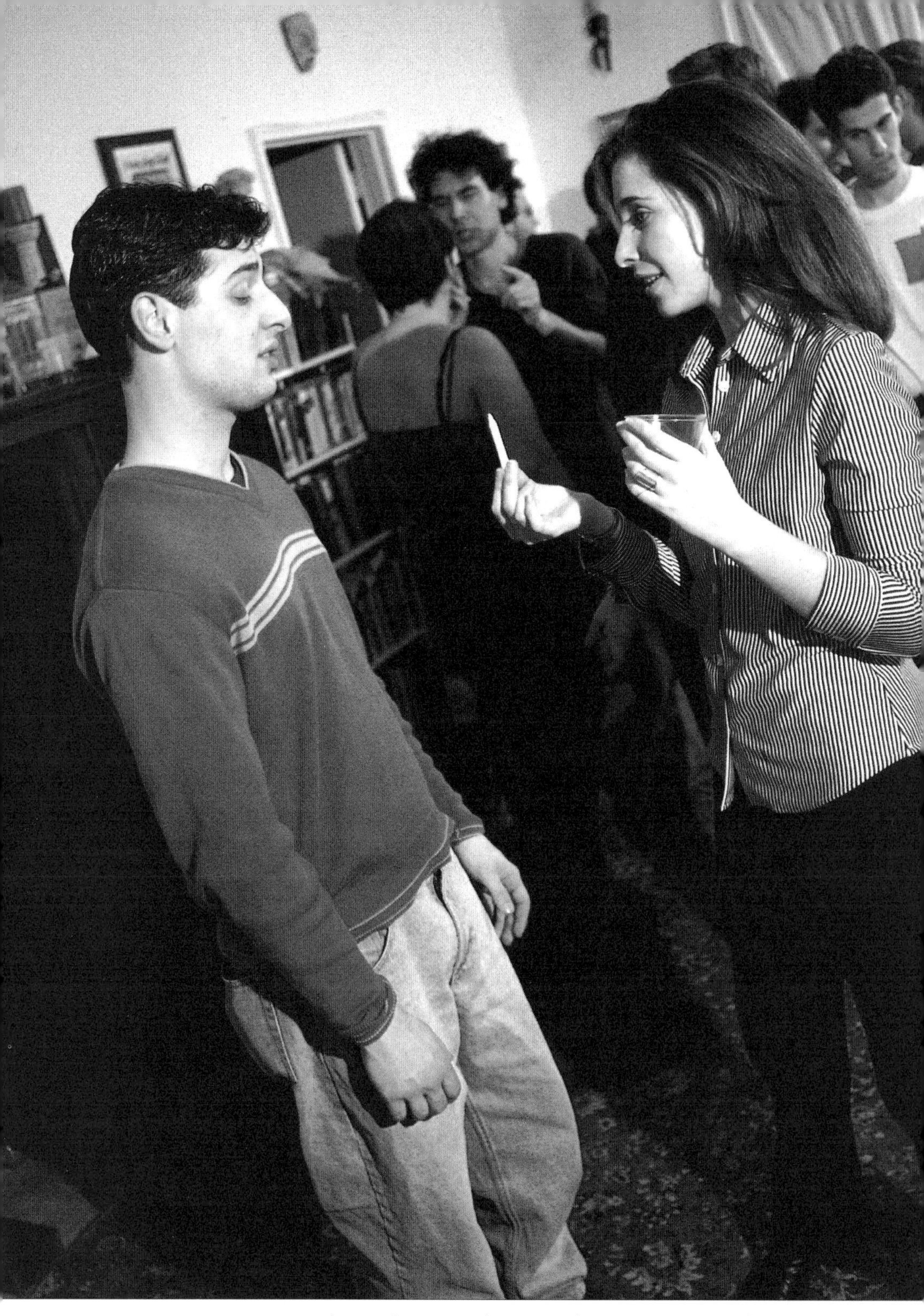

You never know for sure what is in the PCP you are taking because it often is mixed with other substances.

THE DRUG ABUSE PREVENTION LIBRARY

PCP: HIGH RISK ON THE STREETS

Jennifer Croft

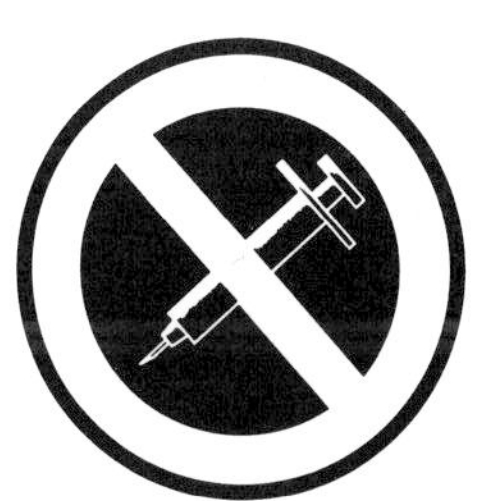

THE ROSEN PUBLISHING GROUP, INC.
NEW YORK

Published in 1998 by The Rosen Publishing Group, Inc.
29 East 21st Street, New York, NY 10010

First Edition

Library of Congress Cataloging-in-Publication Data

Croft, Jennifer, 1970-
PCP / Jennifer Croft.
p. cm. -- (The drug abuse prevention library)
Includes bibliographical references and index.
Summary: Examines the harmful effects of PCP abuse and addiction and explains the dangers of teenage drug use in general.
ISBN 0-8239-2774-1 (lib. bdg.)
1. Phencyclidine abuse--Juvenile literature.
1. Phencyclidine. 2. Drug abuse.] I. Title. II. Series.
RC568.P45C76 1998
362.29'4--dc21 98-13882
CIP
AC

Manufactured in the United States of America

Contents

Introduction

Troy was at his friend Raymond's house after school. The two boys were in Raymond's living room watching television when Raymond's mother came home from work. Troy knew that she was a doctor at a busy hospital and usually didn't come home until late at night.

Raymond's mother poked her head into the room. "Hi guys," she said. "I'm home early because there was a little accident at the hospital."

"Okay," Raymond said, his eyes on the TV set. But as his mother entered the room, what he saw shocked him. Mrs. Navarro had a bandage over her nose, and her eye was badly bruised.

"Mom! What happened?" Raymond cried.

Mrs. Navarro sank down onto the couch. "It was pretty scary," she said. "A guy who was wacked out on drugs came into the emergency room. It took five of us to restrain him. I'm pretty sure it was PCP. These cases are pretty easy to spot."

"Why are they easy to spot?" Troy asked.

"Someone on PCP feels no pain," Mrs. Navarro explained. "And they feel like they have superhuman strength. Sometimes they hallucinate, too. They don't even realize they're hurting themselves and other people."

PCP, or phencyclidine, is not new to the drug scene. Nor is it a particularly popular drug among illegal drug users these days. However, this substance is still a danger to anyone who uses it and the people who come in contact with them.

Angel dust is the most common street name for PCP. But a person on PCP is far from angelic. PCP can make users unpredictable and violent.

This book will provide you with important information about PCP and its dangers. You will learn about this drug's history and about its effects. Even though PCP is not currently a popular street drug, drugs go in and out of fashion. Becoming informed about PCP is an important step in protecting yourself from this drug's harmful effects.

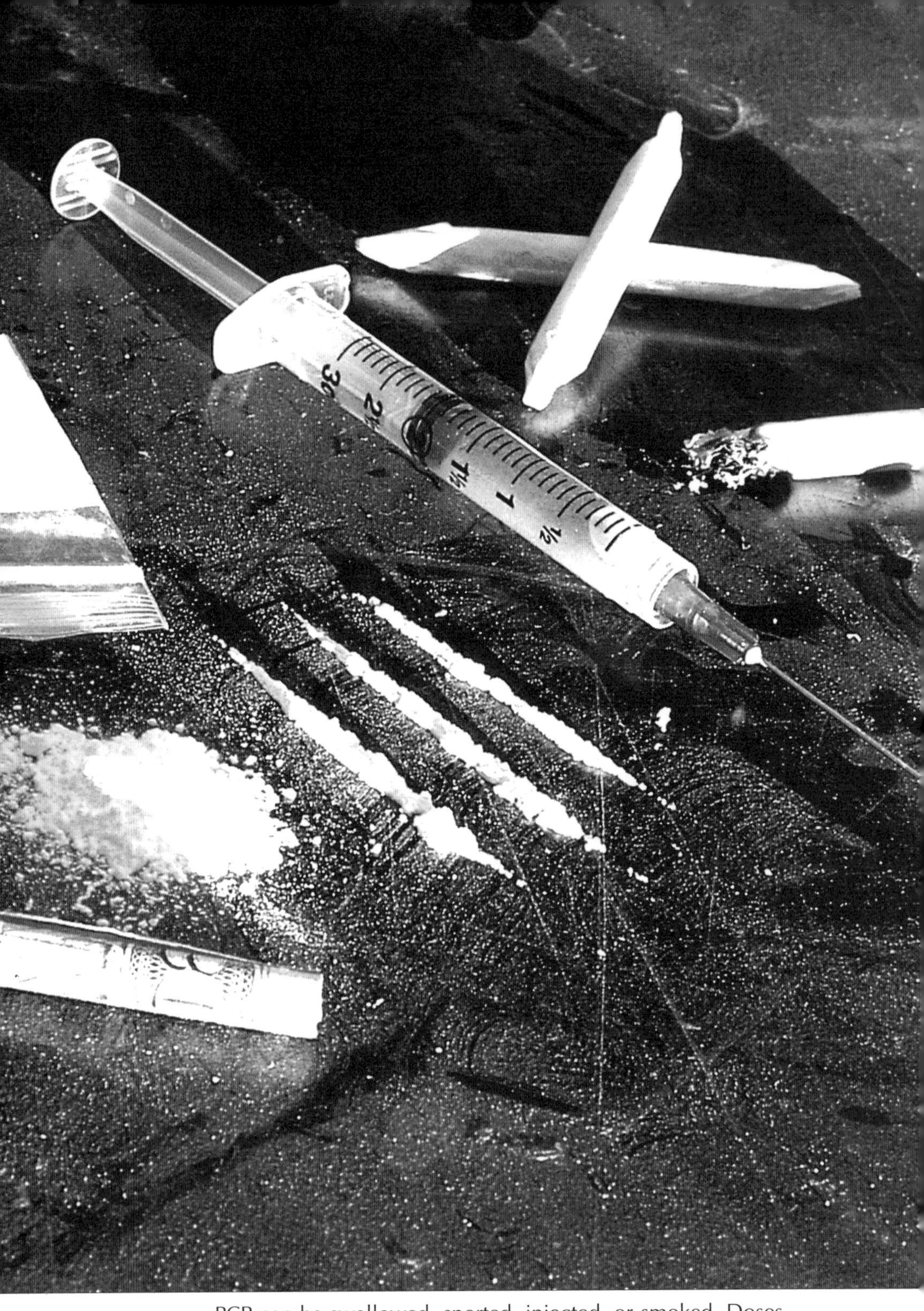

PCP can be swallowed, snorted, injected, or smoked. Doses vary in strength, so it's hard to know how much you are taking.

CHAPTER 1

What Is PCP?

Jacinta started dating Richard during her junior year of high school. Richard had already graduated, and his lifestyle seemed exciting to Jacinta. He always knew of a lot of parties going on around town, and he seemed to have tons of friends. One Friday night, Richard took Jacinta to a party at his friend Ben's house. She didn't really know anyone at the party. She just followed Richard around, and he introduced her to people. Someone handed her a beer, and she was so nervous that she drank it quickly. She began to feel more relaxed and started talking to Ben.

"You know, I've got something I think you might like," Ben said to Jacinta. "I scored it yesterday and haven't tried any yet. Are you up for it?" he asked.

Jacinta wasn't sure if she wanted to accept Ben's offer. "What is it?" she asked cautiously.

"Angel dust!" Ben said proudly, taking some capsules from his pocket. "What do you say?" He held one out to her.

Jacinta looked around the room and saw Richard talking to some other friends. She thought about how cool it would be to tell him she had tried angel dust. She was curious about what it would be like. She took the capsule from Ben's hand and swallowed it with the last sip of her beer.

Jacinta talked to Ben some more. After a while he said that he was feeling pretty high and that he was going to go dance. Jacinta told him that she was going to try to find Richard. As she made her way through the crowd, she felt herself getting more and more nervous. She didn't see Richard anywhere. What if he wasn't at the party anymore? Where had he gone?

Jacinta stopped and looked around, confused. People seemed to be bumping up against her, and she elbowed back. "Hey, what's with you?" she heard a girl say angrily, but Jacinta ignored her. She charged through the crowd, feeling frightened and furious at the same time. What if Richard was with another girl, she suddenly wondered. How would she get home?

She turned around and saw Ben behind her. It seemed as if he was following her. Why was he doing that? Jacinta felt her heart racing as she grew more anxious. The crowd of people seemed to be closing in on her. She felt as if she would die if she didn't get out of that house. She thought Ben would catch her and hurt her.

Jacinta was running by the time she got out the front door. She ran into the street, right into the path of an oncoming car.

PCP

PCP is so dangerous and unpredictable that many people who use illegal drugs try to stay away from it. Many people who make the mistake of trying PCP once never want to use it again. Jacinta's feelings of confusion, agitation, and paranoia are typical reactions to PCP. These feelings can distort your judgment and put you in serious danger.

Because of its negative effects, PCP has never been hugely popular among illegal drug users. But it does attract some risk-seekers. The National Household Survey on Drug Abuse stated that, in 1994, 2.8 percent of the U.S. population over twelve years of age reported having used PCP at least once in their lifetime.

PCP probably reached its peak of usage in the mid- to late-1970s. In 1979, 7 percent of high school seniors had used

PCP in the previous year. In 1995, the number of high school seniors reporting PCP use had dropped to 1.8 percent.

While this seems to show that fewer people are using PCP today, an alarming article in the September 1996 issue of *Teen* magazine stated that "angel dust is making a comeback."

Between 1993 and 1994, the number of high school seniors who had used PCP in the last month rose from .1 percent to .3 percent. About one-third of high school seniors surveyed in 1993 believed that PCP was "fairly easy" or "very easy" to get.

Recognizing PCP

PCP is illegally manufactured in secret labs. Unlike drugs such as cocaine, heroin, and marijuana, which are derived from plants, PCP is entirely artificial. It is made from industrial chemicals.

PCP is a white crystalline powder that dissolves in water and alcohol to become a clear, yellow, or tan liquid. Sometimes it is mixed with dyes and is sold as a colored powder. It is also sold in the form of tablets and capsules. PCP has a very bitter chemical taste.

Neighbors complaining of a terrible chemical smell often alert police to illegal PCP labs. PCP labs also have a tendency

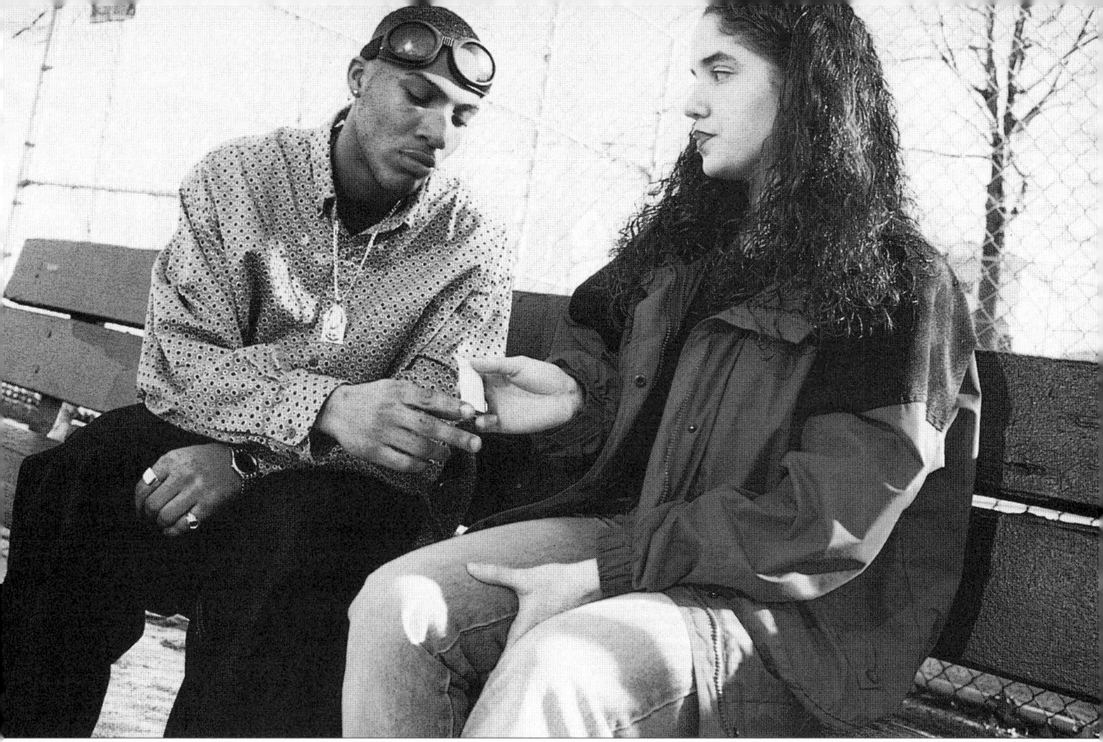

PCP is not as common as many other drugs, but its use has increased among teens.

to catch fire because the "chemists" mixing the drug do not handle the dangerous chemicals properly.

PCP can be swallowed, snorted, injected, or smoked. Most often, it is smoked. When PCP is smoked, it is often applied to a leafy plant such as mint, parsley, oregano, or marijuana, which is then rolled into a cigarette paper. Or, regular cigarettes are dipped in PCP and smoked. Children have become severely ill and even died from inhaling the second-hand smoke of people smoking PCP.

You can't trust drug dealers to sprinkle PCP evenly on a leafy substance like marijuana. There is no way to know whether you are getting a deadly dose of PCP. Two out of three people who end up in hospital emergency rooms after bad PCP reactions say that they smoked PCP that had been sprinkled on another substance.

Sometimes "magic" mushrooms (psilocybin) are soaked in PCP and eaten. A less common way to take PCP is to place the liquid directly into the eyes with an eyedropper. Liquid PCP is so potent that it can be absorbed directly through the skin.

No one, not even experts, can identify PCP by sight. It must be chemically tested. Sometimes dealers will try to pass PCP off as mescaline, peyote, or another drug. The user, anticipating the less intense high provided by another drug, is not prepared for the feeling he or she gets from PCP. This element of surprise can contribute to an even more extreme reaction to PCP.

Dangerous Doses

Even when users know that they are buying PCP, there is no way for them to be sure how much PCP they are getting. The Addiction Research Foundation in Canada analyzed street samples of PCP and found that the PCP content ranged from 1.3 to 81 milligrams per unit dose.

A first-time user might take a weak dose of PCP and not experience a strong reaction.

He or she might take a larger dose the next time, thinking this will increase his or her reaction to the drug. If the PCP content happens to be very high, the combination of a larger dosage and stronger content can result in overdose or death.

Any method of taking PCP is risky, but injection is the most dangerous way. If you inject too much of a substance, it is very difficult for your body to remove it from your system. Injecting drugs is also very dangerous because shared needles can pass on HIV, the virus that causes AIDS, and other serious diseases.

Because PCP can be added to other drugs without the user's knowledge, it is better to avoid any kind of drug use. Any size dose of PCP can cause a violent reaction. Marijuana or "magic" mushrooms may contain PCP and can have much more serious effects than you ever expected. Also, a person who takes PCP for the first time without realizing it is likely to have a bad reaction. One bad reaction to PCP, sometimes called a bad trip, increases your chances of having them in the future.

Street Names

It is especially important to be aware of street names for PCP. It comes in so many

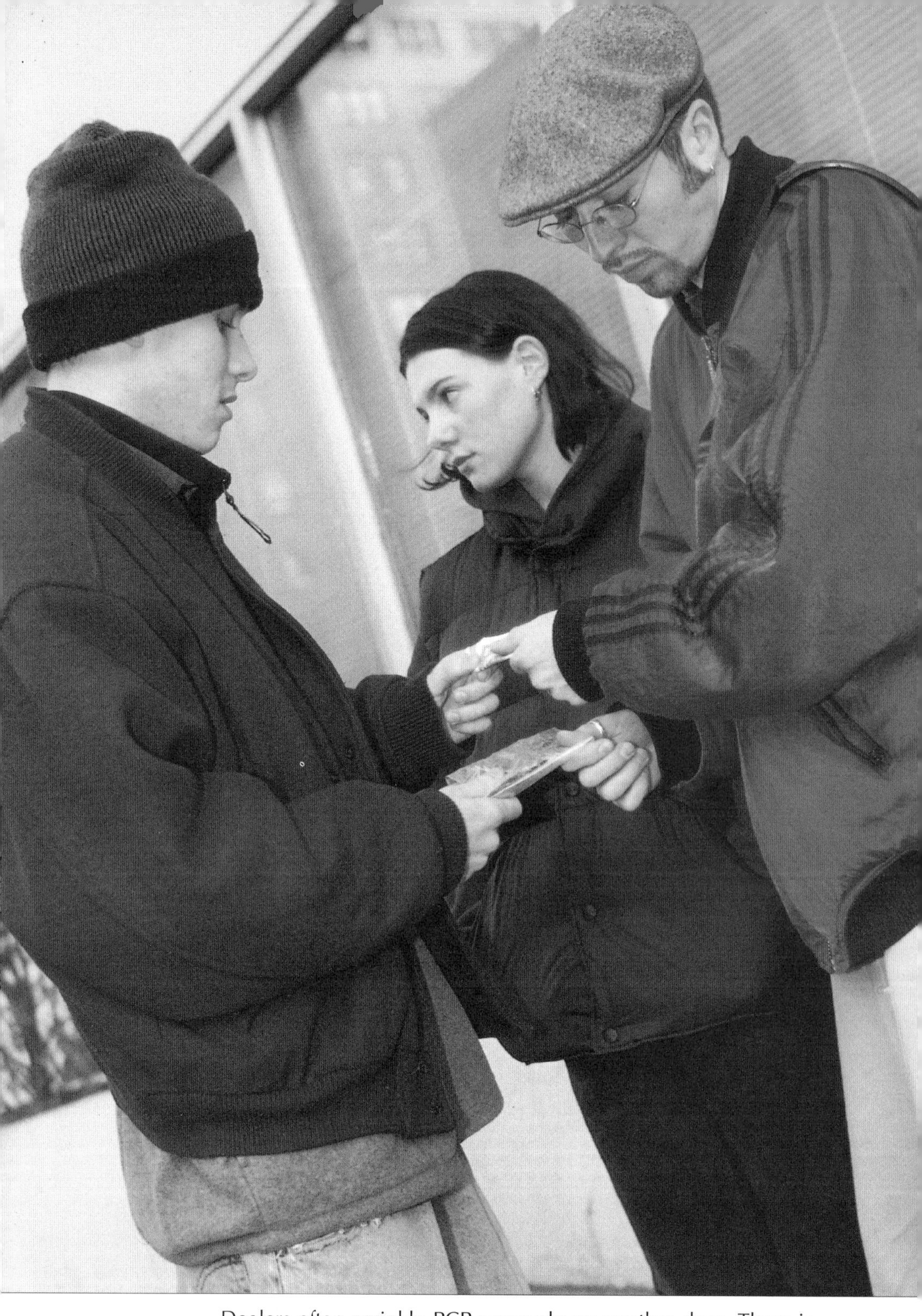

Dealers often sprinkle PCP unevenly on another drug. There is no way to know if you are getting a deadly dose.

forms that it may be difficult to identify. In addition to angel dust, other street names for PCP include ozone, wack, rocket fuel, peace, krystal, angel poke, dummy dust, cluster, clickum, clicker, love, and sherms.

Other street names, such as trank, monkey dust, pig killer, horse tracks, elephant, and gorilla biscuits, refer to PCP's origins as an animal tranquilizer. Still other street names seem to refer to PCP's unpredictable effects: crazy coke, crazy eddie, mean green, madman, butt naked, energizer, embalming fluid, killer, lethal weapon, and devil's dust, for example.

There are also various street names to describe a mixture of PCP and other substances. Some of these refer to the fact that drug dealers often sprinkle PCP on marijuana or other substances. These names include crystal supergrass, killer joints, super kools, mint weed, zombie weed, super joint, wobble weed, magic dust, and dusted parsley.

Beam me up Scottie, clicker, and space base are terms for PCP mixed with crack. Peanut butter means PCP mixed with peanut butter, and octane is PCP mixed with gasoline. Black acid is PCP mixed with LSD.

The History of PCP

PCP was first developed in 1958 as an anesthetic to use on people during surgery. However, patients showed signs of being agitated, irrational, and even psychotic after their operations. Doctors concluded that PCP was not a safe anesthetic for humans. In 1965, they stopped using PCP on humans. Veterinarians then used the drug, under the trade name Sernyl, as an anesthetic for large primates. However, veterinarians no longer use PCP today either.

The federal government classifies drugs by different "schedules." Drugs are classified according to their potential for abuse and their possible medical use. PCP is a Schedule I drug, which means that it has no acceptable medical use and has a high potential for abuse. Schedule I drugs are illegal to manufacture, sell, or consume in the United States. When the government put PCP on Schedule I, illegal labs began making and selling it.

PCP's first appearance as a street drug occurred in 1967 at a rock music festival in San Francisco's Golden Gate Park. A group of people who had made PCP illegally in underground secret labs came to the festival and passed out free samples to musicians and fans. They called the drug they handed out "the PeaCe Pill." Many people had severe reactions to the drug and had to be rushed to a nearby medical clinic. PCP was not an instant favorite among drug users. Its effects scared many people.

For the next ten years, PCP was often passed off as another drug or mixed with another drug. In the mid-1970s, however, PCP made a comeback. The media closely covered its rising popularity. It was a source of great concern among citizens and law enforcement officers alike. It became known that PCP was a very unpredictable drug. It could make users extremely violent, or it could have an opposite effect. It could make them act like zombies.

PCP has become less popular since the 1970s, mostly due to its frightening effects. In the next chapter, we will look more closely at these effects.

CHAPTER 2

The Effects of PCP

Rahmel's brother Corey had started hanging out with a new group of friends. Unlike his old group of friends, these guys weren't interested in sports or music. As far as Rahmel could tell, Corey's new friends were only interested in one thing: drugs. When Rahmel came home from baseball practice, he could hear Corey and his friends in the basement talking and laughing loudly. Corey made sure that his friends were gone by the time his and Rahmel's parents came home.

Rahmel noticed that, on those evenings, Corey acted strangely after his friends left. Sometimes he would be hyperactive, loud, and funny and would keep the family entertained. Other times he skipped dinner and just went to his room and shut the door. Rahmel knew that drug use probably

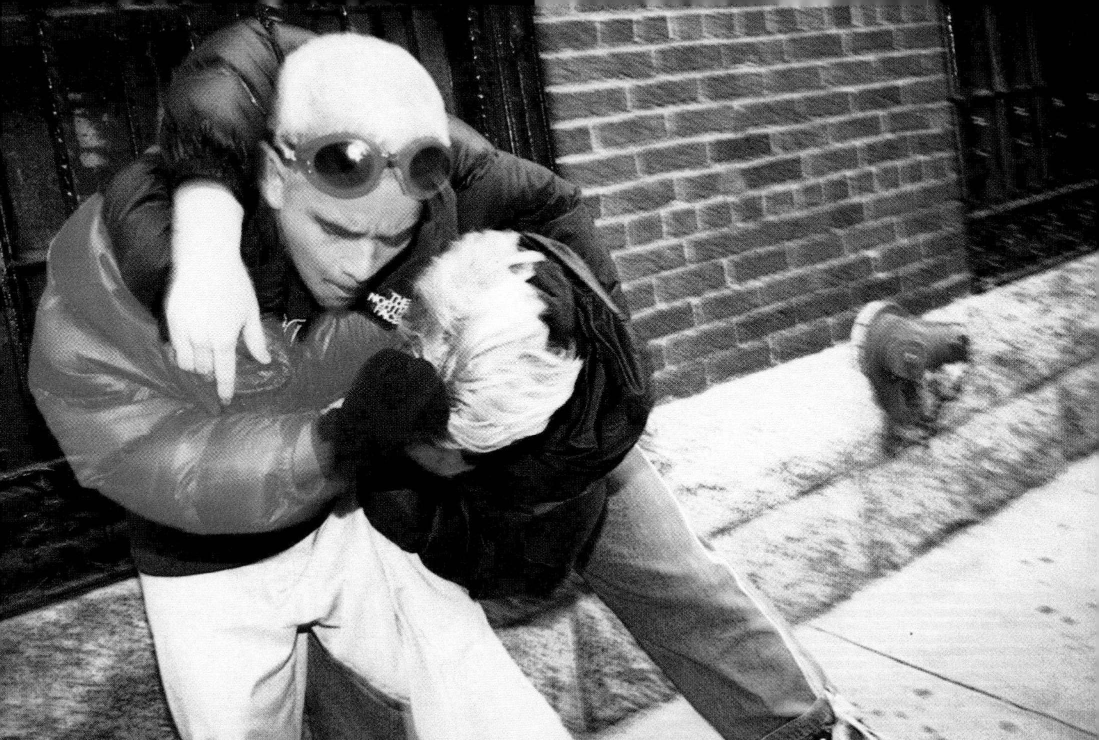

You can become very violent under the influence of PCP.

caused Corey's strange behavior, but he didn't want to tell on his brother. He hoped his parents would notice that Corey was not acting normally, but they often got home from work very late or seemed too tired or busy to notice that anything was wrong.

One night after Corey had spent the afternoon in the basement with his friends, he came into the living room where Rahmel was watching television. Corey walked over to the couch, picked up the remote control from the armrest, and changed the channel.

"Hey, what are you doing? I was watching that!" Rahmel said angrily.

Corey suddenly threw the remote at Rahmel, barely missing his brother's head. "So change it back if you want," he said.

Rahmel was startled by his brother's action and decided to leave him alone. He got up and started to walk out of the room. Corey suddenly attacked him from behind and threw him down on the floor. Rahmel was younger than his brother, but he was bigger and stronger. He fought to get Corey off him. But Corey was pummeling him with his fists and somehow managed to keep Rahmel pinned to the floor.

Rahmel didn't want to hurt his brother, but he didn't want to get himself hurt either. He started throwing punches back. They didn't seem to have any effect at all on Corey, who just kept fighting.

The boys' mother came home and found them struggling on the floor. She yelled at them and tried to pull Corey off Rahmel, but Corey knocked her down. "Mom, call 911!" Rahmel managed to yell. His mother crawled over to the phone. When the police came, it took four officers to restrain Corey and handcuff him. They took him to the emergency room, where the doctors told their mother that Corey had been high on PCP.

PCP and Your Body and Mind

What does PCP do to your body and mind? Why does PCP scare even experienced drug abusers?

The effects of PCP can be very different from one person to another. They even differ from one dose to another for the same person. PCP does not fit easily into one drug category. Depending on how much you take, PCP can act as a stimulant (a drug that speeds up the body's functions), a sedative (a drug that makes the user relaxed), a hallucinogen (a drug that makes the user see and hear things that are not really there), or all three.

PCP is usually classified as a hallucinogen. A hallucinogen is a drug that distorts your perception of reality. Perhaps the best-known hallucinogen is LSD (lysergic acid diethylamide), also known as acid. Hallucinogens affect your senses of direction, distance, and time. They can cause you to see things that aren't there and to behave in ways that you normally wouldn't.

Remember, PCP was first developed as an anesthetic. Even though hospitals no longer use PCP, it still numbs a user's sense of pain. This is very dangerous because, under the influence of PCP, you may hurt yourself or others and not even realize it. PCP also has strange effects on muscular ability. Users become stronger than they normally are. Again, this can make them very dangerous.

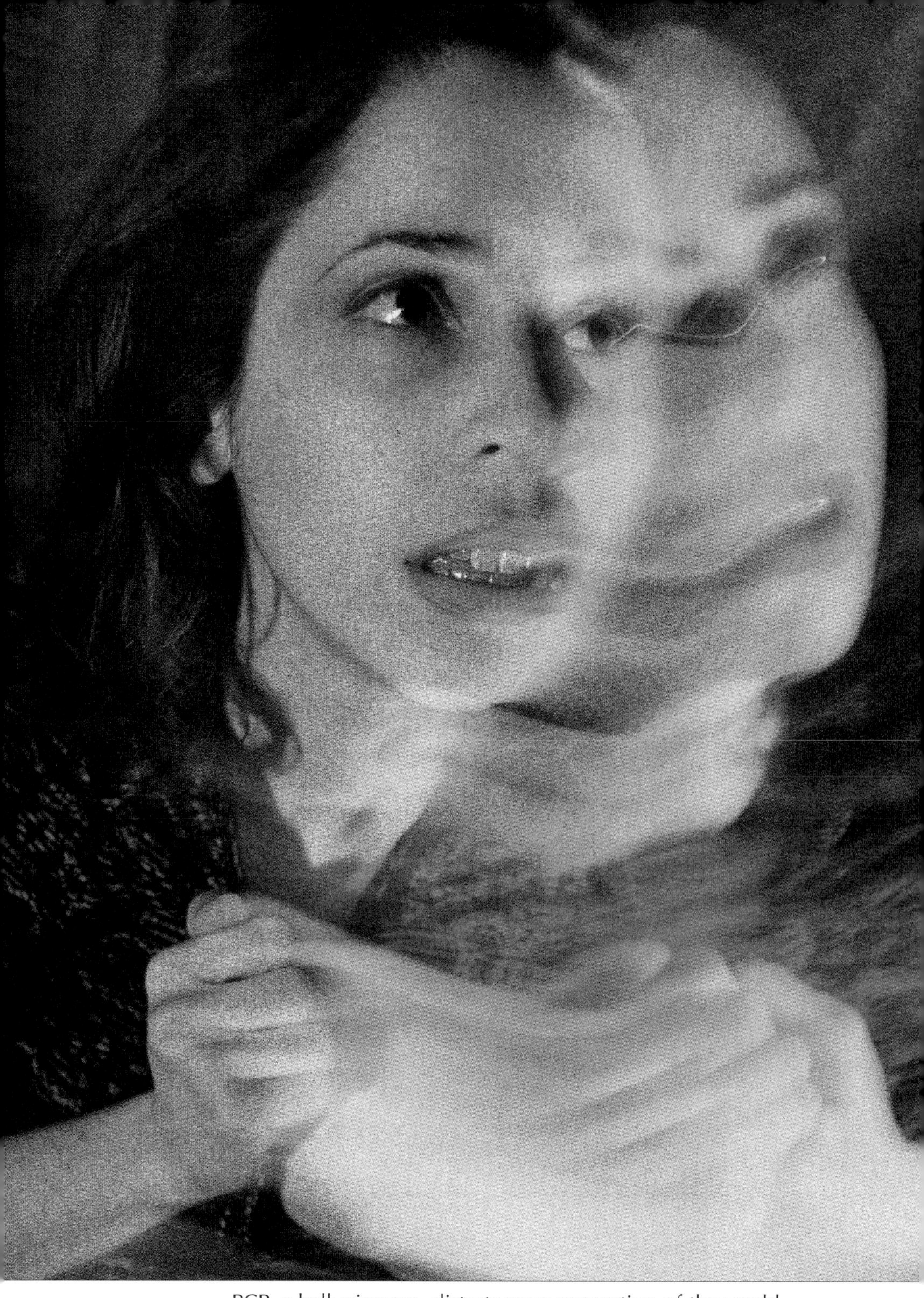

PCP, a hallucinogen, distorts your perception of the world around you.

Danger Signs

In lower doses, the effects of PCP include:

- increase in breathing rate, blood pressure, and pulse rate
- shallow breathing
- heavy sweating
- numbness of hands and feet
- poor muscle coordination

In higher doses, the effects of PCP include:

- drowsiness
- decrease in breathing rate, blood pressure, and pulse rate
- nausea and vomiting
- blurred vision and involuntary eye movement
- drooling
- loss of balance and dizziness
- garbled speech
- symptoms similar to schizophrenia (delusions, sense of distance from one's environment)
- coma
- death caused by repeated convulsions, heart and lung failure, or the rupture of blood vessels in the brain

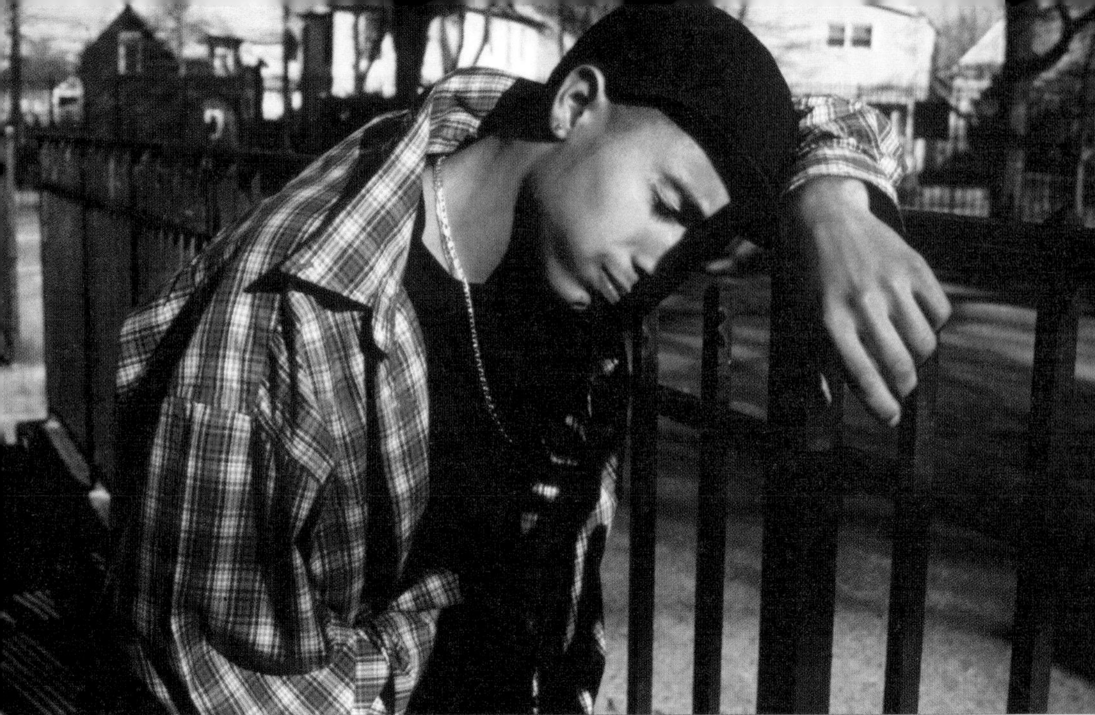

PCP can remain in your body for months after you use it, causing long-term side effects.

Long-Term Effects

The body can store PCP for a long time. It stores PCP in the liver, lungs, brain, and fat cells. PCP may remain in your body's fat cells for months and can be reabsorbed into your blood. This means that even months after you take PCP, you may still experience side effects. It can take as long as one year for PCP to leave the bodies of people who have used it heavily. Stress or exercise can cause PCP to be released from the fat cells where it has been stored.

Regular PCP use can negatively alter users' memory, perception, concentration, and judgment. Long-term users say that they sometimes have difficulties with memory and speech. They sometimes even hear sounds or voices in their heads.

The effects of PCP are cumulative. Users who have taken several small doses may experience the same horrible side effects as a person who has taken one large dose. There is no safe way to experiment with PCP.

PCP causes long-lasting numbness in many parts of the body, including the lungs. The normal body response to the presence of smoke and dirt particles in the lungs is to cough. However, when someone is on PCP, the lungs do not react normally, and the user does not cough. This can lead to a buildup of foreign matter in the lungs and eventually to lung disease and lung tissue damage.

PCP use can be especially harmful to teenagers, because it may interfere with hormones related to normal growth and development. The effects of PCP on the brain—such as short-term memory loss—can seriously damage your ability to learn properly.

PCP and Birth Defects

PCP can hurt unborn children. If a pregnant woman takes PCP, it can affect her baby's blood pressure and heartbeat. The baby's body is unable to get rid of the PCP.

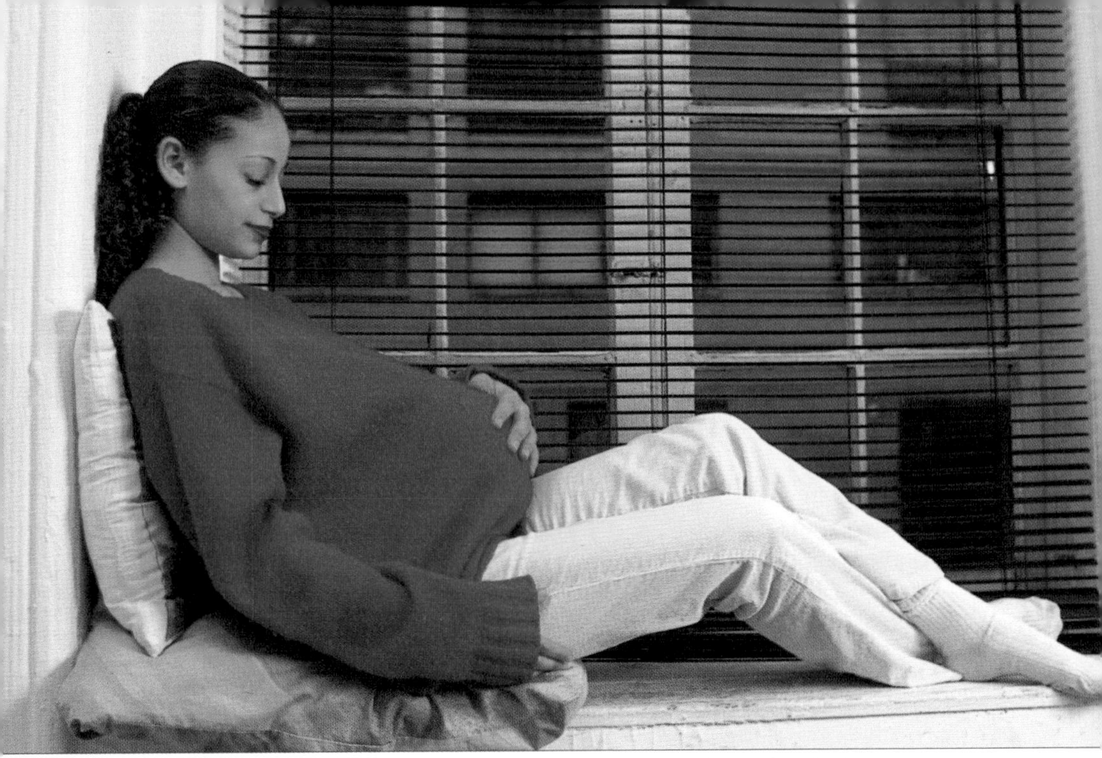

If a pregnant woman takes PCP, it can harm her baby.

Babies who have been exposed to PCP in the womb are often more irritable than other babies. Their faces and bodies may twitch and shake uncontrollably. Still, it is uncertain whether PCP causes long-term mental damage to children who are born with PCP in their systems.

A mother also can pass PCP to her baby through breast milk. Studies on rabbits and mice have found that PCP is ten times more concentrated in the mother's breast milk than in the mother's own blood. Another study on rats found that PCP affects the brain of the fetus more than the brain of the mother. When a pregnant woman puts PCP into her body, she is putting it into her unborn baby as well.

PCP Psychosis

In her book *Angel Dusted: A Family's Nightmare*, Ursula Etons tells the true story of her son Owen's struggle with PCP. Owen was a student at college when he suddenly began behaving very strangely. He had to return home from college in the middle of the year so his family could take care of him. His doctors concluded that his behavior was the result of having taken PCP. Owen had gone into a PCP psychosis, and it took many months of treatment before he could function normally again.

A PCP psychosis is a temporary mental disturbance caused by PCP. The psychosis affects the user's thought processes. A person experiencing a PCP psychosis may show many of the same symptoms associated with schizophrenia. He or she is detached from reality. It can be impossible to communicate normally with someone in a PCP psychosis. A PCP psychosis may last for days, weeks, or months after the person has taken PCP. During this time of mental instability, a person is at high risk for committing suicide.

CHAPTER 3

Terrifying Trips

Pam and Diana were roommates in college. They didn't know each other before they came to school, but they soon became close friends. They both liked to go to parties and meet guys. Pam and Diana were excited about a big party on Saturday night. The party was at the fraternity house that was supposed to have the best-looking guys. The girls spent most of Saturday getting ready for the big night. When the bouncer let them in the door at the party, they congratulated themselves, deciding that it must be because they looked so good.

The frat was packed with people. Pam and Diana got drinks and wandered around the house. Two guys named Gregg and John approached them. The four of them talked for a few minutes, and then Gregg suggested that they all go up to the roof. "It's a lot quieter up

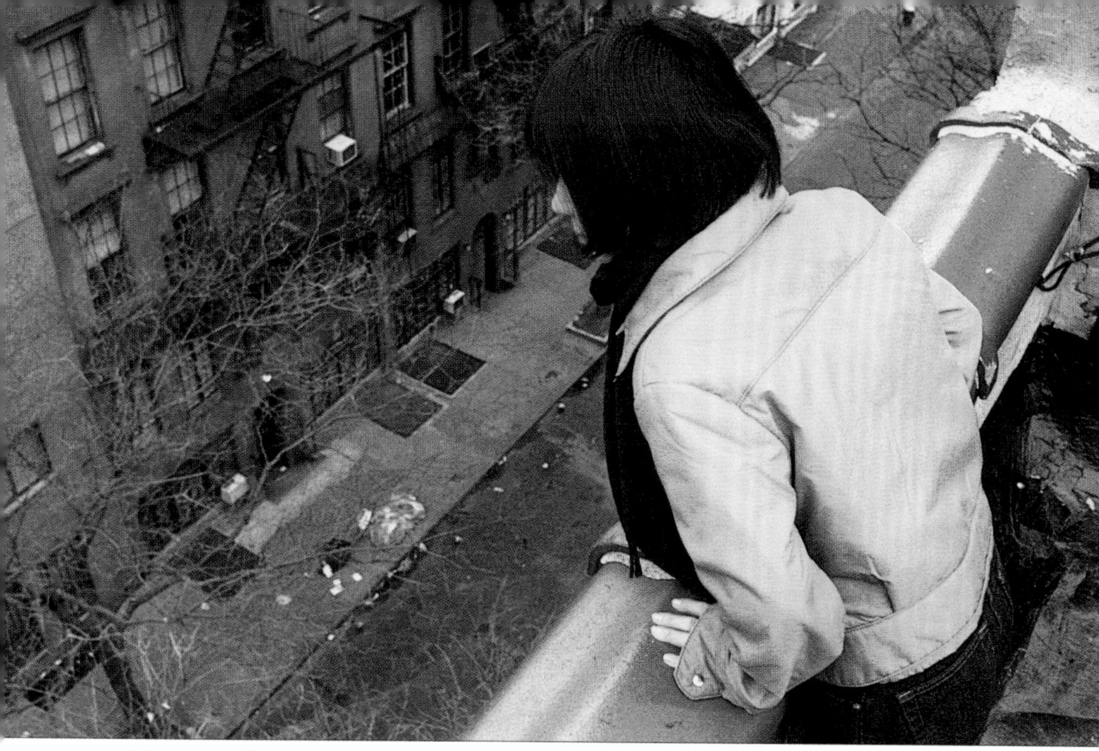

PCP can affect your perception of distance. It can make things appear closer than they actually are.

there, and we can check out the stars," he said. Everyone agreed that it was a good idea.

Once they were up on the roof, Gregg and John both lit up joints and offered some to Pam and Diana. The girls were nervous about smoking pot, but neither wanted to seem like a nerd. They each took a joint and started smoking it. After the four of them had finished smoking, Pam turned to Diana and whispered, "I don't feel anything. Do you?" That's when she noticed that Diana looked as if she was going to be sick. "Hey, are you okay?" Pam asked, concerned.

Diana shook her head. "I feel so weird," she said. "Everything looks weird. I feel like I'm floating in space, and you're all really far away." Then she looked over toward the edge of the roof. "What's that?" she said, pointing at the house next door. "I want to go over there."

"What are you talking about?" Gregg said. "You can't get there from here. Are you sure that you're okay?" But Diana didn't answer. She walked over to the edge of the roof and climbed onto the ledge. "I can make it from here!" she shouted back at them.

"What are you doing? Stop! Diana!" Pam cried out. She stood frozen in horror. The guys weren't moving either.

"No, I know I can do it!" Before anyone could stop her, Diana leapt off the ledge toward the other house. She fell four stories. Pam, Gregg, and John ran over to the edge of the roof and looked down at Diana's lifeless body on the pavement.

Lab results showed that the joint Diana had smoked had been dipped in PCP. The drug had made her think she could jump from one roof to the other. John told the police that he didn't know the pot had been mixed with PCP. After all, he, Gregg, and Pam had not gotten laced joints. But that didn't make Pam feel any better about losing her best friend.

Dangerous Behavior

Many kinds of drugs—both legal and illegal—are dangerous and have negative side effects. PCP is even more dangerous

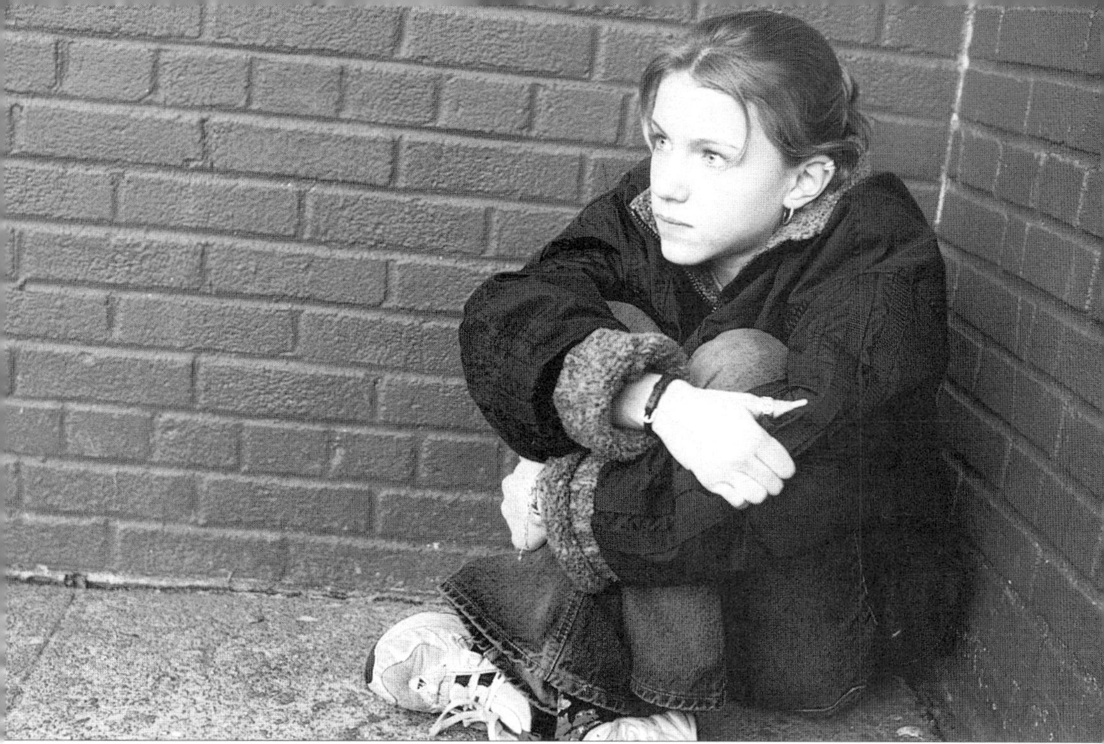

PCP is unpredictable. It affects different people in different ways.

than most drugs. If you take PCP, you not only run the risk of having a terrible reaction to the PCP itself, you also take the chance that the PCP will cause you to do something to injure or even kill yourself. The National Institute on Drug Abuse reports that PCP causes violence or agitation in one-third of the people who use it.

You have already read that people on PCP can behave in bizarre and violent ways. This behavior makes them a danger to themselves and others. Users usually do not remember their behavior while they were high on PCP. Under the influence of PCP, they become delusional. They are convinced that their warped perceptions are real.

In one grisly case in New York state, two teenage boys on PCP gouged out another boy's eyes and stabbed him to death. They mistakenly thought that he had stolen some of their PCP.

PCP users may bite themselves, stand naked outside in cold weather, or exhibit other strange, self-destructive behaviors. There have also been many reported cases of people on PCP who have broken out of handcuffs or continued to attack someone even after being shot or stabbed many times. On PCP, users do not feel physical pain in the way that they normally would. They can exhibit extraordinary strength and endurance.

A person on PCP may believe that his or her body parts actually belong to someone else. For example, a PCP user may think that his own injured, bleeding arm is actually someone else's arm. He doesn't realize that he himself is injured.

PCP users are at great risk for car accidents, drownings, fights, and other kinds of dangerous consequences. These include climbing up to high places or jumping out of windows.

PCP affects different people in different ways. Its effect depends on how someone takes the drug, how much of it he or she takes, whether he or she takes it with another drug, the purity of the PCP, and the body chemistry of the user. Mixing PCP with other drugs, like alcohol, cocaine, or heroin, can be deadly. The Drug Abuse Warning Network reports that five out of six people who die with PCP in their bodies were taking at least one other drug.

PCP Look-Alikes

Because illegal labs manufacture PCP, there is no way for a user to know whether he or she is taking pure PCP. People who buy what they think is PCP may be placing themselves in great danger because of the many PCP analogs (look-alikes) on the street. Chemists easily play with the formula for PCP to create other drugs with similar effects. Analogs of illegal drugs are called "designer drugs."

Sometimes illegal labs try to create analogs because they may be cheaper, more potent, or more difficult to detect than the drug that they are designed to replace. However, these drugs are still illegal. According to a federal law passed in 1986, synthetic analogs of illegal drugs are illegal to possess, sell, or manufacture. Designer drugs can also be deadly. The so-called chemists at illegal drug labs can easily make mistakes and create lethal concoctions. Don't believe anyone who tells you that a new designer drug will give you a PCP high without side effects. There is no way to know if you're getting a "safe" drug.

At least 125 analogs for PCP have been identified. Some of the street names of PCP look-alikes are PCE, PHP, PCPP, TCE, and TCP. One study found that PHP was actually becoming somewhat more popular than PCP because it is more difficult to detect in the user's body. Sometimes ketamine, an animal tranquilizer known on the street as "Special K," is also substituted for PCP.

PCP and Its Effect on Society

Because PCP users present grave danger to themselves and others, the drug has an extremely negative effect on the rest of society. People on PCP are not safe on the road nor in any other public place. People on PCP have hurt and even killed innocent people. PCP users who end up in emergency rooms cost the health care system money and take doctors' valuable time away from other patients. PCP also places a greater burden on the law-enforcement system.

Strangely, some good may come from PCP. In the 1970s, the huge increase in emergency-room patients with PCP reactions led

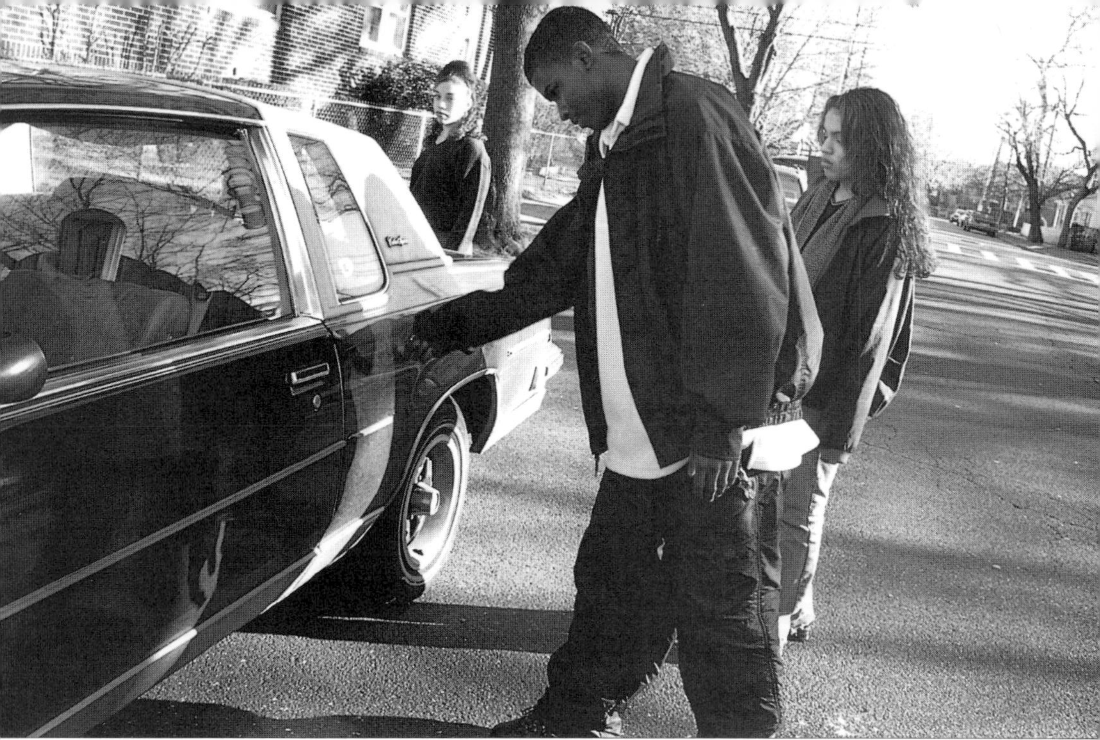

A driver on PCP is a danger to himself and his passengers, as well as to other drivers and pedestrians.

many hospitals to develop drug abuse intervention programs.

More recently, the effect of PCP on the brain is being carefully studied by scientists who believe that this research may help people who have problems related to the brain. For example, the way PCP reacts with the chemicals in the brain is helping scientists to determine the cause of schizophrenia. Due to studies of the way that PCP affects brain activity, research may also be able to help people who suffer from strokes, heart attacks, and other traumas.

PCP can be a helpful tool to scientists studying these problems, but it is doubtful that they will use PCP again medically. PCP has too many harmful side effects.

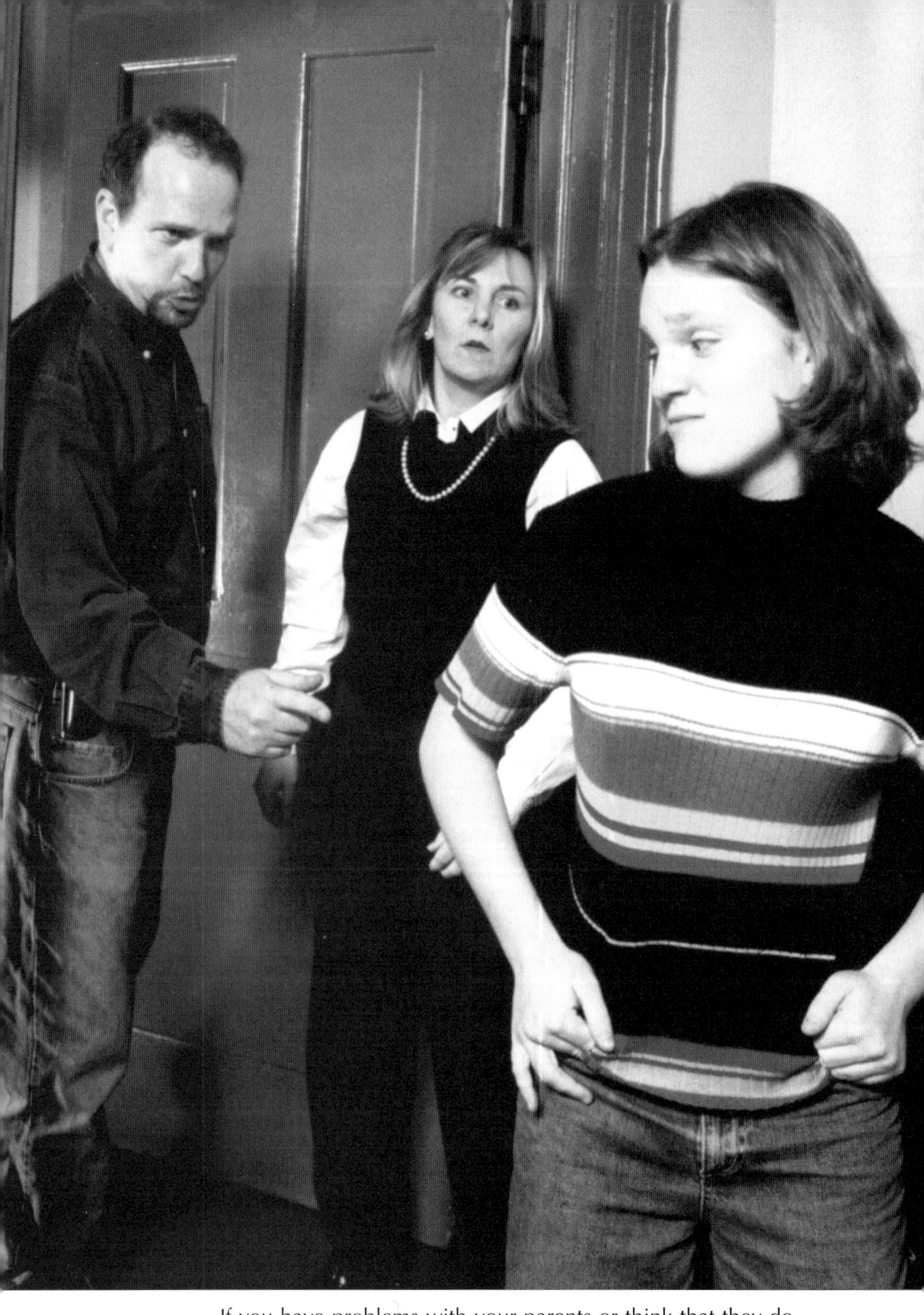

If you have problems with your parents or think that they do not understand you, taking drugs will only make matters worse.

CHAPTER 4

PCP Abuse and Addiction

Shira had always been known as a daredevil. Even when she was a little kid, she would do crazy, silly things. As she got older, her stunts became less innocent. Sometimes she and her friends sneaked into the public pool at night and drank beer. Other times they shoplifted from stores. Shira was always looking for the next big adventure. If there was danger involved, she wanted to do it. That's why it wasn't hard for a dealer to persuade Shira to try "killer weed"—marijuana joints that had been dipped in PCP.

Everyone else in Shira's group of friends was too scared to try the killer weed. Shira jumped at the opportunity. She liked how the drug made her feel. She felt powerful and invincible when she did it. The drug made her feel as if she could do anything. Shira started smoking killer weed regularly. Then she started snorting PCP. She felt as if she had found the drug that best fit her personality.

One day, the police arrested Shira's drug dealer. The police in her town were cracking down on drugs, and Shira couldn't find anyone who would sell her PCP. After a few days of not taking the drug, Shira craved the high she got from PCP. She tried to forget about the cravings. Soon, however, she couldn't ignore the way she was feeling without the drug. She was in a bad mood all the time. She felt nervous and anxious. She slept terribly and woke up during the night with chills and diarrhea. All she could think about was when she could get more PCP.

The Path to Addiction

Why do people take PCP? It is a relatively cheap drug, and it is often easily available. Sometimes PCP attracts teens because of its unpredictable effects. To them, PCP offers a way to do crazy things or have an adventure. Other teens like the way that PCP makes them feel: numb and detached. While they are on PCP, they don't feel or care about anything. They may think that PCP helps them to express anger and even rage. PCP also has a reputation for erasing painful memories.

Many teens abuse PCP for the same reasons that they abuse other drugs. Peer pressure is a major factor in teen drug use. Research has shown that teens usually overestimate how many of their peers are using drugs. Because they think so many other teens are doing drugs, they may feel embarrassed about not using drugs also. This may make them more susceptible to peer pressure.

Teens may also take drugs because of boredom or a desire to try new things. Finally, they may want to rebel against the authority figures in their lives, such as teachers and parents.

The Facts About Addiction

Addiction occurs when a user needs a drug to feel normal. The user's body and mind become dependent on the drug.

Evidence shows that PCP users can become chemically dependent on the drug. This means that their brain chemistry changes and they can no longer feel good without PCP. They can also become psychologically dependent on the drug, meaning that they start to crave its effects.

In one study, monkeys who were given PCP for one month showed signs of physical withdrawal when researchers suddenly stopped giving them the drug. Their withdrawal symptoms included diarrhea, chills, drowsiness, and teeth-grinding.

Babies born with PCP in their systems also experience withdrawal symptoms. They may be jittery, irritable, have high-pitched cries, and have difficulty nursing.

People who have become dependent on PCP and stop taking the drug experience withdrawal symptoms. These symptoms can include:

- depression
- poor memory
- confusion
- flashbacks
- headaches
- increased need for sleep
- craving for PCP

The unpleasantness of withdrawal often causes users to take PCP again. In one study of emergency-room patients with PCP in their bodies, most patients said they had taken PCP because they were dependent on it.

Because withdrawal can be a painful experience, it can be difficult for users to quit on their own. Medical professionals can help addicts to cope with the process

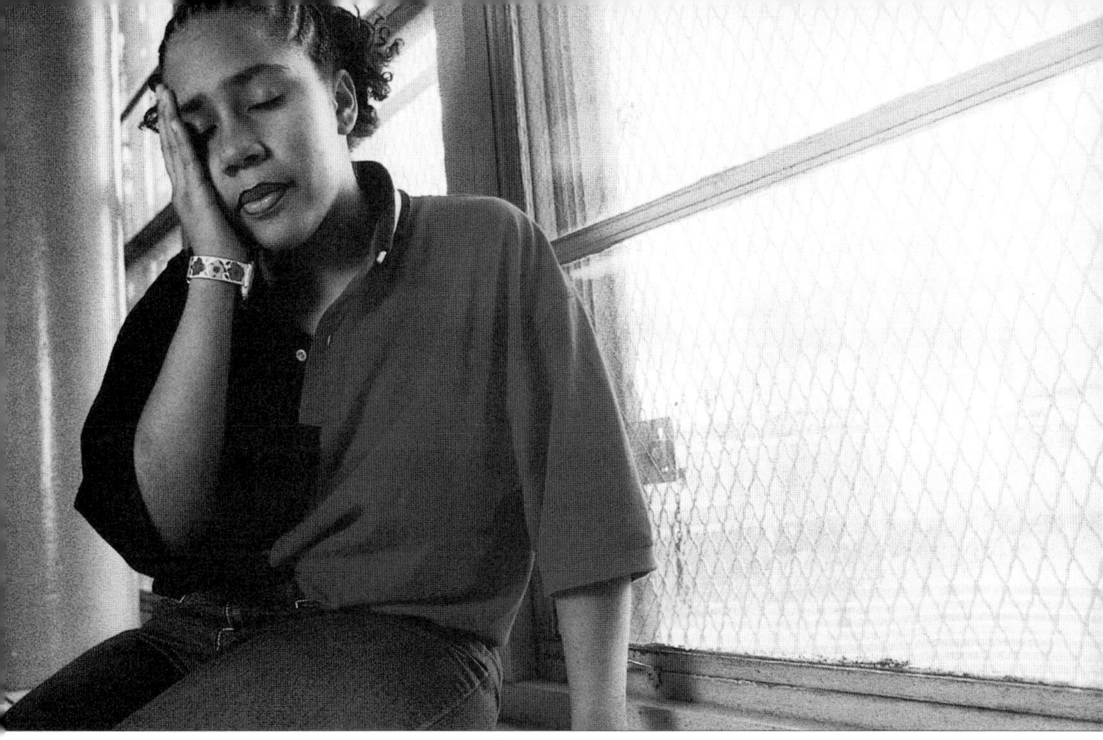

Withdrawal is a painful process. Headaches are a common symptom of withdrawal.

of withdrawal. Also, addicts often need professional help to understand why they have made drugs a part of their lives. For most addicts, therapy is essential for recovery.

Shira's parents noticed her strange behavior and her physical symptoms. They spoke with their family doctor, who had known Shira since she was a baby. Dr. Wenger suspected that Shira might be going through drug withdrawal. Her suspicions were confirmed when Shira's parents brought Shira in for a checkup. Shira confessed that she had been taking PCP and was now suffering because her supply had been cut off.

"Taking PCP again will make you feel better right now, but that's not the solution,"

Dr. Wenger said. "We need to get you into a rehabilitation program so you won't need PCP in your life anymore."

Rehab wasn't easy, but Shira stuck with it. Dr. Wenger referred her to a therapist who helped Shira work out her problems with her parents. Through therapy, Shira began to see how she had been using PCP as an excuse to continue to be wild and daring, when in reality she was frightened about the path her life was taking. Therapy helped Shira to realize that it was okay to grow up and not be a crazy kid anymore. She began to appreciate her own courage and assertiveness, and she learned to channel those qualities in more productive and useful ways.

CHAPTER 5

Preventing PCP Abuse

Chris had always been a shy, quiet kid. In elementary school, other kids picked on him because he was so soft-spoken. As he grew up, Chris continued to feel insecure. He never felt like he fit in. Even in high school, people still picked on him all the time.

Chris got an after-school job at a music store. That's where he met Molly. They both loved music, and they both hated high school. Chris and Molly started spending time together after work. Sometimes they even skipped school to hang out. Molly introduced Chris to some great new bands. She also introduced him to PCP. Chris had never tried drugs, but Molly was his first girlfriend. He really wanted her to like him, so he agreed to try PCP.

One night after Molly and Chris took PCP, they decided to crash a party some of the jocks were having. Before Molly knew what was happening, Chris had started a fight with some of the guys who used to make fun of him. Nobody had ever seen him so aggressive and angry. They couldn't hold him back.

Chris liked the way that PCP had made him feel powerful. It made him want to take PCP more often. But his behavior had scared Molly. She told him to quit or she would break up with him. Chris chose PCP over Molly.

A few weeks later Chris was in the hospital for slamming his fist through a window while on PCP. He told a social worker at the hospital about his problem. She helped him get into a drug treatment program. It wasn't easy, but Chris kicked his drug problem. It made him realize that he really was a strong person. He saw that he didn't need PCP to make himself feel powerful anymore.

Spotting a Drug Problem

The National Clearinghouse on Drug and Alcohol Information has compiled a list of signs that indicate someone may have a drug problem. You can look for these signs in yourself or someone you know. Be aware if a friend exhibits one or more of the following behaviors:

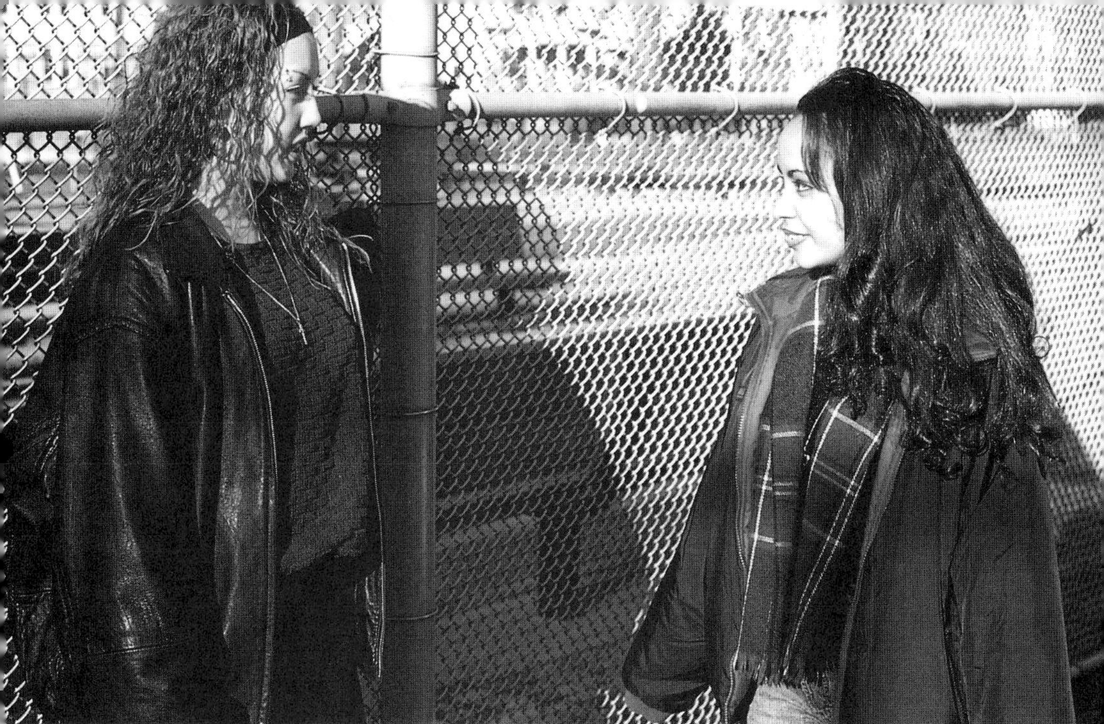
If someone you know is taking PCP, talk to them about it and encourage them to seek help.

- Getting high on a regular basis
- Lying about things, for example, how often they are using drugs
- Avoiding others to get high
- Giving up activities they used to do, or friends who don't do drugs
- Having to use more and more of a drug to get the same effect that they used to experience using smaller doses
- Constantly talking about drugs
- Believing they need drugs to have fun
- Pressuring others to do drugs
- Getting in trouble with the law
- Taking unnecessary risks
- Feeling depressed, hopeless, or even suicidal

- Being suspended from school for a drug-related incident
- Missing work or school because of drugs

If you believe that someone you know is taking PCP or other drugs, and you feel comfortable talking to the person about it, tell them that you are worried about them. Encourage them to seek help. Be a supportive friend. If that doesn't help, or if you don't feel as if you can talk to the person directly, speak with a trusted adult. This person can be a parent, family friend, neighbor, teacher, doctor, counselor, religious leader, social worker, boss, or coach. You don't have to solve the problem on your own.

There are also warning signs to look for in yourself if you think you might have a drug problem (or even if you don't think you do). If one or more of these statements are true for you, it may be time to seek help.

- You cannot predict whether or not you will use drugs;
- You believe that in order to have fun you need to use drugs;
- You have trouble at work or school because of drug use;
- You turn to drugs after an argument or confrontation to relieve your uncomfortable feelings;

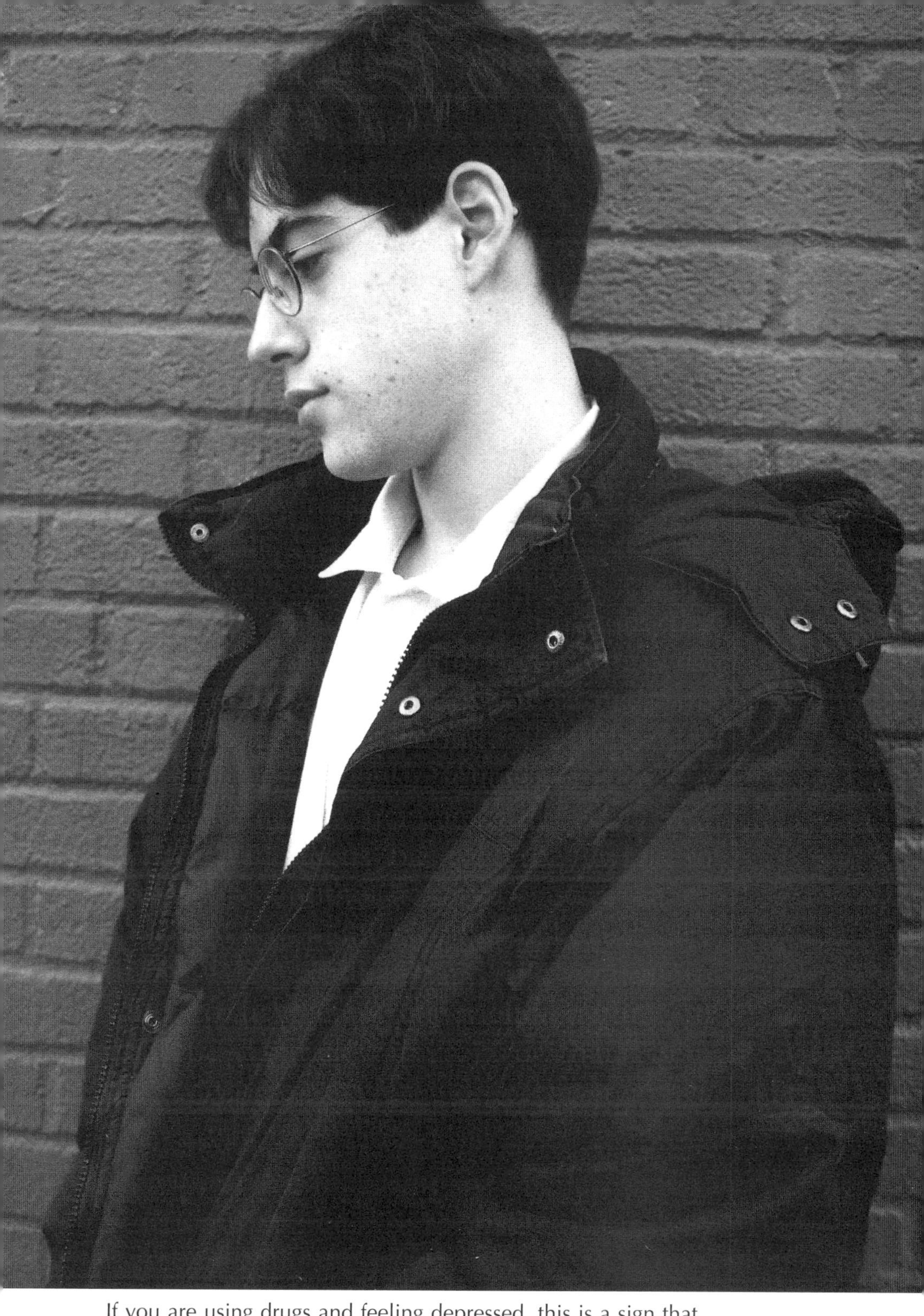

If you are using drugs and feeling depressed, this is a sign that you may have a problem.

- You use more drugs to get the same effect you once got with smaller amounts;
- You use drugs alone;
- You don't remember how you have behaved after you have used drugs;
- You make promises to yourself or others that you'll stop using drugs, but you are unable to keep them;
- You feel alone, scared, miserable, or depressed.

How Do You Know If Someone Is on PCP?

It can be difficult to tell if someone you know is taking PCP. The effects of PCP vary from person to person, and even from dose to dose. There is no single sign that indicates PCP use. However, bizarre or violent behavior may be an indication of PCP use. Other symptoms to watch for are drowsiness, sweating, drooling, vomiting, poor coordination, slurred speech, and involuntary eye movement.

What to Do If Someone Has a Bad Trip

If you are with someone who has a negative reaction to PCP, your quick thinking can save them (and others) from serious harm.

First, the person should be in a quiet, calm environment, such as a dim room without windows. Make sure that he or she is not near moving vehicles, in a public place, or in a high place such as a rooftop. Don't try to restrain the person physically. This can cause them to become violent.

Call 911 as soon as possible. An experienced professional may be able to "talk down" the person having a bad trip. In many cases, a person on PCP needs sedative drugs to restrain him or her. Cranberry juice can help to acidify the urine and remove PCP from the body faster.

A person experiencing a negative reaction to PCP may be totally out of control. The person may hurt you even though you are good friends. Watch out for your own safety too.

If You Have a Problem with PCP

If you have abused or are addicted to PCP or other drugs, you have taken a major step by picking up this book. You have read how dangerous PCP can be. If you take PCP, it is important to stop. Using PCP puts you and others at great risk. It is also illegal.

If you are addicted and can't stop taking PCP on your own, talk with an adult you trust about getting help. If there is no one you feel comfortable talking with, call one of the toll-free numbers listed at the back of this book. You will not have to tell the counselor your name. You can also look in the phone book under the words Drug Abuse or Drug Addiction.

Among the services you may find listed are community drug hotlines, local emergency health clinics, community treatment services, city or local health departments, hospitals, and other groups such as Narcotics Anonymous.

It can be difficult to talk to your parents about drugs, but you will need their emotional support if you go through the treatment process.

Even if you are not addicted to PCP or another drug, it can be helpful to talk to a counselor about why you want to experiment with drugs. Often people turn to drugs for reasons that have nothing to do with the drugs themselves. You may want to examine your life and consider why you feel the need to escape through drugs.

Resisting Peer Pressure

If your friends are pressuring you to take drugs, you can use what you have learned in this book to say no. Nobody has the right to make you do something that puts your

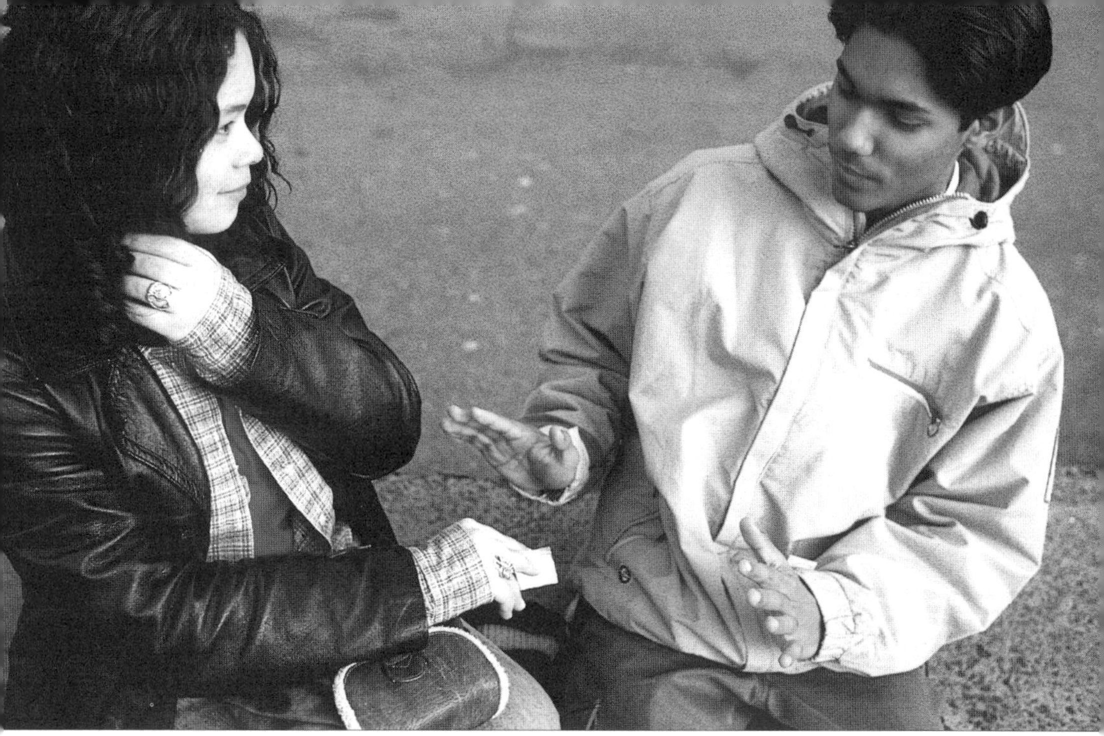

You can say no to friends who are pressuring you to take drugs. No one has the right to make you put yourself at risk.

health—and even your life—at risk. The person who pressures you to take PCP or other drugs doesn't really care about you.

Remember, too, that it's always harder to be the one who sticks out from the crowd than the one who goes along with everyone else. Your friends will respect you more for taking a position that is important to you. They may even follow your lead.

Sometimes hallucinogens like LSD and PCP attract teens because they want to experience another reality. They've heard stories of how hallucinogens make ordinary things look extraordinary. It's natural to want to have new experiences, but you don't need to risk your life to do that. There are ways to explore different realities without drugs. Playing virtual-reality or computer games, watching movies, acting, reading, and even traveling to a new place are some examples of ways you can experience new things.

There's nothing wrong with wanting to escape reality once in a while. But if you feel a strong, persistent need to escape from your life, you should discuss this with a parent, another trusted adult, or a telephone counselor.

Some people like that PCP makes them feel strong and powerful. However, these feelings are artificial. The sense of strength people get from PCP isn't real strength. If you want to try PCP because you feel weak or helpless, it's important to realize that PCP will cause more problems than it solves. Again, counseling can help you to examine your feelings and help you to gain more control over your life. An important step in taking control of your life is refusing to let PCP be a part of it.

Glossary

agitation A state of being easily excited or upset.

AIDS (Acquired Immunodeficiency Syndrome) An almost always fatal disease that attacks the body's immune system. There is no known cure for AIDS.

analog Something that is similar in function to something else, but has a different origin.

anesthetic A drug or other substance that causes total or partial loss of physical feeling.

convulsion An intense, uncontrollable muscular contraction.

crystalline Made up of crystals or resembling crystals.

cumulative Building up over time.

delusion False belief.

detached Uninvolved emotionally or socially.

flashback A vision of the past that one has usually suddenly and very clearly.

hallucinogen A drug that alters a user's perception of reality, causing him or her to see things that are not there.

HIV (Human Immunodeficiency Virus) The virus that causes AIDS. HIV can be contracted through the exchange of bodily fluids, such as blood, semen, or vaginal fluids.

irrational Unreasonable.

lethal Deadly.

mescaline A drug that produces hallucinations and which is derived from the mescal cactus.

paranoia An unreasonable feeling that others are out to get you.

peyote Another term for the mescal cactus, from which a hallucinogenic drug is derived.

phencyclidine The chemical name for PCP.

potent Powerful, strong.

psychosis A severe mental disorder in which the victim loses touch with reality and cannot function normally.

psychotic The kind of behavior caused by psychosis.

rehabilitation A program to help someone recover from drug abuse or addiction.

schizophrenia A mental disorder characterized by a withdrawal from reality and severe mental disturbance.

secondhand smoke Smoke inhaled by a person who is not smoking, but is near a smoker.

susceptible Sensitive, vulnerable.

synthetic Artificial, human-made.

withdrawal The often painful process that occurs when a person stops taking a drug to which he or she has become addicted.

Where to Go for Help

American Council for Drug Education
164 West 74th Street
New York, NY 10023
(800) 488-DRUG
Web site: http://www.acde.org

Center for Substance Abuse Prevention (CSAP)
5600 Fishers Lane
Suite 800, Rockwall II Building
Rockville, MD 20857
(301) 443-0365
Web site: http://www.samhsa.gov/csap/index.htm

National Clearinghouse for Alcohol and Drug Information
P.O. Box 2345
Rockville, MD 20847-2345
(800) 729-6686
(301) 468-2600
Web site: http://www.health.org
e-mail: info@health.org

National Council on Alcoholism and Drug Dependence (NCADD)
12 West 21st Street
New York, NY 10010
(800) NCA-CALL (622-2255)
(212) 206-6770
Web site: http://www.ncadd.org
e-mail: national@NCADD.org

National Drug Information Treatment and Referral Hot Line
(800) 662-HELP (4357)

National Families in Action
2296 Henderson Mill Road, Suite 300
Atlanta, GA 30345-7239
(770) 934-6364
Web site: http://www.emory.edu/NFIA/

National Institute on Drug Abuse (NIDA)
Public Information Department
5600 Fishers Lane, Room 10A39
Rockville, MD 20857
(800) 729-6686
Web site: http://www.nida.nih.gov
e-mail: information@www.nida.nih.gov

In Canada:

Addictions Foundation of Manitoba
1031 Portage Avenue
Winnipeg, MB R3G 0R8
(204) 944-6200

For Further Reading

Carroll, Marilyn. *PCP: The Dangerous Angel*. Solomon H. Snyder Ed. New York: Chelsea House, 1991.

Clayton, Lawrence. *Designer Drugs.* Rev. ed. New York: Rosen Publishing Group, 1998.

Hurwitz, Sue and Nancy Shniderman. *Drugs and Your Friends.* Rev. ed. New York: Rosen Publishing Group, 1995.

Landon, Elaine. *Hooked: Talking About Addiction.* Brookfield, CT: Millbrook Press, 1995.

McCormick, Michelle. *Designer-Drug Abuse.* New York: Franklin Watts, 1989.

Newman, Gerald and Eleanor Newman. *PCP*. Springfield, NJ: Enslow Publishers, 1997.

Seymour, Richard, et al. *The New Drugs: Look-Alikes, Drugs of Deception, and Designer Drugs.* Center City, MN: Hazelden Foundation, 1989.

Stafford, Peter G. *Psychedelics Encyclopedia.* Berkeley, CA: Ronin Publishing, 1992.

INDEX

About the Author

Jennifer Croft is a graduate student in international relations and a freelance writer. This is her second book about teenagers and drug abuse. She lives in Boston, Massachusetts.

Photo Credits

All photos by John Bentham